CALMING YOGA
for mental and spiritual well-being

Darlene Graham Stanisiewski

*The mission of Storey Publishing is to serve our customers
by publishing practical information that encourages personal independence
in harmony with the environment.*

Edited by Deborah Balmuth
Cover design by Wendy Palitz
Cover illustrations by Alexandra Eckhardt and Alison Kolesar
Interior illustrations by Alison Kolesar
Text design and production by Susan Bernier

Copyright © 2002 by Storey Publishing, LLC

All rights reserved. No part of this book may be reproduced without written permission from the publisher, except by a reviewer who may quote brief passages or reproduce illustrations in a review with appropriate credits; nor may any part of this book be reproduced, stored in a retrieval system, or transmitted in any form or by any means — electronic, mechanical, photocopying, recording, or other — without written permission from the publisher.

The information in this book is true and complete to the best of our knowledge. All recommendations are made without guarantee on the part of the author or Storey Publishing. The author and publisher disclaim any liability in connection with the use of this information. For additional information, please contact Storey Books, 210 MASS MoCA Way, North Adams, MA 01247.

Storey books are available for special premium and promotional uses and for customized editions. For further information, please call Storey's Custom Publishing Department at 1-800-793-9396.

Printed in the United States by Lake Book
10 9 8 7 6 5 4 3 2 1

ISBN 1-58017-892-8

Table of Contents

Introduction: A Path to Reducing Stress • 2

Calming the Mind
with Simple Meditation • 7

Beginning Your Yoga Practice:
Warm-ups • 15

Standing Poses • 31

Floor Stretches • 47

Recommended Reading • 62

Introduction:
A Path to Reducing Stress

I would like to share with you how yoga became important to me as I embarked on my spiritual path. At the age of 41 years I became interested in learning how to meditate. I began to open up to the possibility of using meditation as a way to steady my mind and soothe my spirit. A good friend of mine took me to a meditation center where I tried to meditate; however, I had trouble sitting still without discomfort in my body. At that time, I did not know that what I was experiencing was the effects of stress on my body. As a nurse, my conditioned response was that something had to be wrong with my body for me to have so much pain while sitting.

My friend, Andy, had been taking yoga classes at the time and thought yoga would be helpful to me. When he showed me a few postures, I immediately knew that yoga was for me. I began taking classes with Linda Smith, who lived in Hadley, Massachusetts, at the time, and from there my yoga practice started to be an important part of my life. Soon, I

Benefits of Yoga

* Increased sense of well-being
* Increased flexibility and strength
* Calming of the mind and body
* Integrating and honoring of all the organs of body/mind

was led to the Kripalu Yoga Center in Lenox, Massachusetts, where I continued my journey. Within a few years, I became connected with the Northampton (Massachusetts) Yoga Center owned by David Garlock, who now lives in New York. With David's inspiration and support, I started a teacher's training course at his center in 1995. As a result, much healing has taken place in my body and mind. My allergies and other stress-related ailments have improved as I continue on this journey of healing.

So I invite you to let go of any preconceived ideas about yoga and let this experience be a gentle mothering of your body, your mind, and your spirit — whatever that is for you.

Cautions Before You Begin

As you embark on the practice of yoga, it is important to honor the limits of your body. Do not start this practice if you have had any recent bone or muscular injury, if you have untreated hypertension (high blood pressure), or if you are pregnant, unless you have your doctor's permission. And remember — you are your own expert, and you must use your own wisdom as you enter into the practice of yoga.

I also want to stress how important the warm-ups are; they are a way to warm the muscles and help yourself feel a deeper release.

Finally, there will be some days when you will feel more rigid and less open. Honor that feeling, and do not force your body to do what is uncomfortable.

To love oneself is the beginning of a lifelong romance."

— Oscar Wilde

Calming the Mind with Simple Meditation

Calming the mind and tuning in to the subtle energy of "Prana" or "Chi" within our bodies enhances healing and reduces stress. Yoga (the word means union between mind and body) is one way to become aware of this healing energy. It is often misunderstood by our fast-paced culture; however, in the past 15 years or so, yoga has become increasingly popular as a way for us to get in touch with our true nature and be healthy and balanced.

Through regular yoga practice, one also becomes aware of many more subtle effects of yoga, such as reducing stress, enhancing the immune system, and calming the mind. As we learn to listen with gentleness and acceptance to what our body needs, a new awareness begins to unfold. The yoga asanas, or postures, help a person become more aware of held tension in the body and of how the mind interprets that tension. The breath, which is an integral part of yoga practice, aids in releasing that tension — as a result, more blood flows and fresh Prana aids in restoring balance. One can feel renewed after a hard day's work with just a few yoga stretches. So I invite you to relax and be open and gentle with yourself as I guide you in preparing for the practice of yoga.

Take a Comfortable Seat

* **Sit in a comfortable position.** If sitting on the floor or in a cross-legged position is too difficult, choose a chair. The important things are that your back is straight, your shoulders are relaxed, and you are not pressuring yourself to be in a position that is uncomfortable.

* **Let all the events from the day** leave your mind, along with any events that you anticipate for the future.

* **Become aware of your breath** without changing it. Notice both the inhalation and the exhalation.

* **Soften your mind and begin to feel** the support of the ground beneath you. If any thought or judgment arises in your mind, just let it be there, and gently come back to your breath.

* **Now imagine a very loving and safe place** where you like to go, whether it be in the mountains, at the ocean, or maybe just in your own yard or garden. Take your time. You have nowhere to go and nothing to do but be with yourself in this loving place.

* **Now bring your awareness to your sitting bones,** and feel the support of those bones as you sit on the earth. Feel the earth holding you.

* **Gently, as you inhale,** begin to press the crown of your head toward the sky. Elongate the the spine, feeling your sitting bones beneath you.

* **Now tune in to the breath once again,** and imagine a balloon in your upper abdomen. As you inhale gently, invite the breath into the balloon and feel the balloon expand as it travels up to your ribs and into your upper chest. Slowly . . . 1 . . . 2 . . . 3 . . . 4.

* **As you exhale, feel the balloon deflate in your upper,** middle, and then lower chest, drawing the muscles of the abdomen in toward your inner spine.

* **Again, slowly inhale** . . . 1 . . . 2 . . . 3 . . . 4. Gently release the muscles surrounding your lower spine while at the same time elongating the spine through the crown of the head.

✳ **As you exhale, count slowly** ... 1 ... 2 ... 3 ... 4 ... 5 ... 6 ... 7 ... 8. Be aware of the sensations in the body, and with the mind of gentleness imagine the breath massaging away any areas of tension.

If you find this difficult to do, then accept whatever thoughts and feelings arise. In the beginning, you may find this simple exercise surprisingly difficult, but with practice and commitment to coming home to yourself, it becomes easier. Just allow yourself to keep an open mind and discover your strengths as well as your limits with kindness toward yourself. Slow down. Listen. Tune in. Breathe. Let go.

Imagine that the breath is kissing your cells to aliveness.

This simple technique of meditation can be practiced both morning and night. In the beginning it might seem like a chore, but as you master the various movements and postures, you will find yourself looking forward to this quiet and relaxing time when you can be with yourself.

 Benefits of Meditation

* Calms the nervous system
* Relaxes the cardiovascular system
* Increases blood flow to the cells
* Strengthens the immune system
* Enhances other forms of exercise

Beginning Your Yoga Practice: Warm-ups

To begin the practice of yoga, you might find it helpful to set aside a space in your home where you will be undisturbed and will be able to be with yourself in a gentle quiet way. A sticky yoga mat (available at yoga studios and supply stores) can help you avoid slipping but is not necessary in the beginning; however, you might eventually wish to purchase one. You may use a folded blanket or a firm cushion to sit on.

Be respectful of and honor the limits of your body. Listen to its wisdom and release learned belief patterns, such as "no pain, no gain." Invite in new concepts, such as "there is strength in gentleness, let that strength come from the inside out." Less is more as you begin to listen and feel your breath opening and releasing held tensions in the body. Let go of any preconceived thoughts of accomplishment and let yourself be in the moment, feeling the sensations in the body. When judgmental thoughts arise, just let them go. Come back to the breath.

Seated Position

Sit in a cross-legged position on a folded blanket or a firm cushion. If you find this position uncomfortable, you may sit with your legs straight out in front of you. Sit close to the edge of the cushion or blanket so that you can let your abdominal muscles relax into the space between your legs. Spread the folds of your buttock muscles so that your sitting bones are firmly planted on the pillow beneath you.

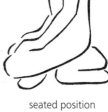

seated position

Gently close your eyes and let your awareness go inside. Notice any sensations you have in the body and gently let them be there without judgment. Now, let go of the events of your day and any plans that you have for the hours or days following this practice, and relax your mind, relax your body . . . let go. Notice your breath without changing it, let it be — just notice. Relax your shoulders.

As you inhale, press down into your sitting bone and at the same time gently press up through the crown of your head. Imagine that the breath is elongating your inner spine, creating space between the vertebrae. Allow your intention to be one of gentleness with yourself.

Neck Stretches

Bring your chin to your chest. Inhale. As you exhale, release into the pull of gravity, letting go. Be aware of the sensations in other parts of the body as well the stretch in the back of the neck. Inhale, lifting your chin but not overextending it, and expand your chest while pressing your sitting bones into the earth. Keep your back straight, gently elongating the spine. Repeat these movements 4 to 5 times.

Breathe.

Bring your head back to center, breathe, and begin to rotate your head from one side of your body to the other without hyperextending your neck. If you should feel any tension in your neck or shoulders, breathe into that place and let the tension go.

Now, roll your shoulders 3 to 4 times from front to back, and then roll 3 to 4 times from back to front. Use your breath to release any held tension.

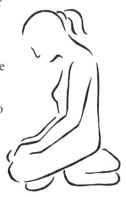

neck stretches

Chest Opener

Place your hands interlaced behind your head. Inhale, pressing your elbows back. Expand your chest, lift your chin — hold — and release, slowly bringing your head forward, keeping your hands interlaced behind your head. Let the weight of your hands guide your body forward, and feel the delicious stretch in your spine and up the back of neck. Breathe. Repeat this movement 4 to 5 times.

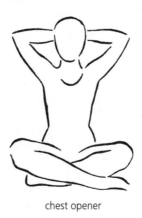

chest opener

Torso Circles

Bring your hands to your knees. Begin to make clockwise circles with your torso, keeping your awareness of the root of your spine, your hips, and your hip sockets. Breathe down into your abdomen, slowly and gently, and let the breath release your lower spinal muscles. As you release the tension commonly held in the hips and lower spine, imagine a fresh supply of blood and oxygen traveling to your abdominal organs and hips. Let the fresh supply of Prana renew your root chakra, the area at the base of your spine.

Pause, breathe, and then reverse direction to make counterclockwise circles.

torso circles

Dog Stretch

Slowly move from a seated position onto your hands and knees (table position). Keep your knees hip-width apart, your hands below your shoulders, palms flat on the floor, and fingers extended and pointing straight in front of you. If your knees bother you, put a blanket under them. Make sure your back is straight. Take a moment to concentrate on your breath. Release into a relaxed back, extending the spine, relaxing the abdominal muscles, pressing the tailbone toward the sky, and extending your neck to look toward the sky. As you exhale, move into the cat stretch (see next page).

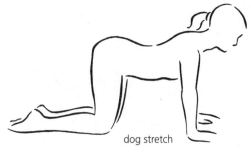

dog stretch

Cat Stretch

As you slowly exhale, tuck the tailbone under; round your back; release your head, yielding to the earth; and contract your abdominal muscles. Hold. As you inhale, go back into the dog stretch (see previous page), and then repeat this inviting stretch sequence 5 times.

Return to the table position, making sure knees are hip-width apart, fingers spread open, palms flat, weight evenly distributed. Again focus on your breath, and take a moment to feel your intention, while tucking your toes under and

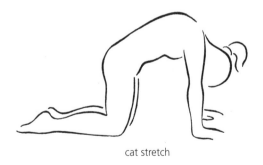

cat stretch

CALMING YOGA | 23

"windshield wipering" your feet side to side. Feel the stretch to the posterior aspect of your toes, making sure that you stretch your small toes as well as your big toes.

Downward Facing Dog

Come back to stillness, breathe down to your abdominal muscles, and begin to press into your hands, while at the same time coming up onto the balls of your feet, with the knees slightly bent.

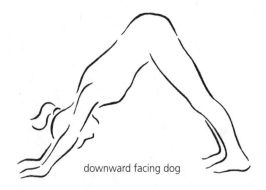

downward facing dog

Press your tailbone toward the sky, elongate the spine as you inhale (creating space between the vertebrae), and press down into the earth as you feel the strength in your arms (without locking your elbows or hyperextending them). At this point your body is shaped like a triangle. You may want to bend the right knee while straightening the left and then vice versa, gently stretching the muscles in the backs of your legs.

Invite the breath in, elongating the spine, and exhale slowly, feeling a slight opening into the stretch, as you begin to press your heels toward the floor. Release your neck and head into the pull of gravity. If you should notice trembling in your arms or legs, do not be alarmed; this is the mind letting go of its grip on the body, to quote one of my Kripalu yoga teachers.

Depending on your flexibility, honor your time spent in this posture. Notice when it begins to feel uncomfortable, and at that point come out of the pose slowly (make these movements a meditation in motion).

Note: If you find downward facing dog too uncomfortable or you are unable to reach the floor, use a solid sturdy chair against a wall. Place your hands on either the back of the chair or the seat, hands shoulder-width apart, feet hip-width apart.

Rag Doll

Walk your feet toward your hands so that you eventually stand in the rag doll position, hands hanging loosely, head

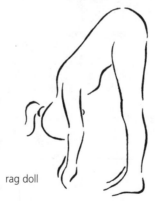

rag doll

hanging, working with gravity. Sway from side to side. Let go of any burdens from the day; breathe and release.

Swaying Side to Side

Inhaling, slowly rise to a standing position, one vertebra at a time, as you exhale.

Stand with your feet slightly more than hip-width apart. Begin to sway from side to side, letting your hands hang loosely. Let your knees be slightly bent as you move gracefully to your right side, then to your left. Let your hands and arms swing out from your body and flop behind you as you move from side to side.

Each time you return to center, inhale, then forcefully exhale as you swing to the opposite side. Let this be a graceful movement; coordinate the breath as you move. Be creative! Let it be like a dance. You might want to come up onto the ball of one foot while you are moving in the opposite direction. Put a spring in your movement. Release any holding of tension in your lower back or shoulders. Coordinate the breath with the movements. Let go!

Chest Opener

Gently, without pushing yourself, come back to stillness and breathe. Interlace your hands at the back of your head (as shown on page 20). Slowly press your elbows toward the wall behind you while elongating the spine, and expand your lungs with a deep inhalation. Next, exhale slowly and bring your chin forward to your chest. Let the weight of your arms gently stretch the muscles at the back of your neck. Let your back round forward; yield to the earth. Breathe in and out.

Slowly return to standing. Inhale while lifting your head and chin, pressing each elbow back, and expand your chest, lift up out of your lower spine, and press into the crown of your head. Repeat this movement 4 to 5 times. On the last repetition, when you round your back, release your hands and let your arms hang forward toward the ground. Sway from side to side. Slowly return to standing as you inhale.

Man is not himself only . . .
He is all that he sees;
all that flows to him from a thousand sources . . .
He is the land, the lift of its mountain lines,
The reach of its valleys.

— Mary Austin

Standing Poses

Mountain Pose

Begin by coming to your usual, everyday standing posture. Just notice and observe whether you stand with feet hip-width apart or closer together. Do you put more weight on one foot or stand on the heels or the toes? Check out your arches: Are they collapsed, or do you have the tendency to tighten your toes? Gently increase your body awareness.

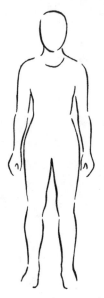

mountain pose

Planting the Feet

Place your feet hip-width apart, heels parallel, feet straight ahead. Begin to gently rock back onto your heels and then forward onto the balls of your feet. Be aware of pressing into the roots of your toes as you come forward. Coordinate the breath with your movement.

After approximately 15 rounds of rocking forward and back, bring your feet back to center and feel the entire soles of your feet connected to the earth. Lift and spread your toes, and be aware of pressing the roots of each large toe and each small toe into the ground. Spread each toe gently on the earth. Feel the balls of each foot firmly planted on the earth. Now, press your heels down and feel your weight evenly distributed on both feet. Lift your arches from both the inside and the outside. Imagine that there are roots growing from your feet into the earth, and feel your firm foundation. Carry this base of support in all your postures.

Scan Your Body

Standing in the mountain pose with your feet firmly planted, scan the lower half of your body. Become aware of your legs and how your feet support your legs. Perhaps one leg might be stronger than the other, and your tendency is to stand with your weight on that leg. Which side do you favor? Notice your knees; do they tend to turn in, or do you tend to hyperextend them? Do you notice any changes in your legs as you work with grounding your feet?

Bring your awareness to your pelvis. What is your habitual posture? Do you tilt your pelvis forward, or do you have the tendency to collapse your lower spine? Just notice. How does your lower body affect your upper body? Usually the tendency is to overcompensate by thrusting the ribs and chest forward or backward.

Return to your awareness of your foundation; breathe into the soles of your feet and feel your weight balanced evenly. Balance your pelvis over your feet, slowly breathe and elongate your spine, press up through the crown of your head. Roll your shoulders up and around in one direction, then the other, and let your arms come rest. Inhale, and lift your knees as you press your feet firmly down to the ground. Feel your upper thigh muscles hugging your thigh-bones. Feel a line of energy traveling down through the core of your legs; feel your strength.

With each breath, elongate your spine, pressing through the top of your head. Now, bring your arms straight out to your sides, turn the palms toward the sky, and continue raising your arms until they are straight over your shoulders and parallel to your ears, palms facing each other. Relax the shoulders at the same time. Practice closing your eyes, being aware of reaching toward the sky and at the same time, pressing into the earth. Imagine yourself as a mountain. Feel your firm foundation and your magnificence. Imagine a line of energy traveling from the crown of your head down through your center to the ground. Be aware of your posture, breathing gently, expanding your chest. Take up lots of room! Point your hands toward the sky while you turn inward and just notice your energy. Stay in this posture until you have reached your toleration point. Do not pressure yourself to stay longer than is comfortable. Release by inhaling, and then slowly exhale, lowering your arms out to your sides. Come to stillness and feel the effects of the mountain pose. Close your eyes; breathe.

Lower-Back Strengthener

Stand in mountain pose with your hands to your sides. Place the palms of each hand, fingers pointing down to the earth, on each side of your lower back, just above your buttocks. Roll your shoulders up and around toward your back while cascading your shoulder blades down your back. Press your hands into the dorsal muscles (the muscles adjacent to your spine). As you press your hands, feel your chest open as you slowly and deeply inhale. Lift your chin as you gaze up; feel your spine lengthening, and energize your legs and feet by pressing down into the ground — hold to the count of 5. Exhale and release. Be aware of all the details as you repeat this posture 5 times.

This posture should feel delicious and pleasurable. If you feel any pain or discomfort at all, quietly return to a place of comfort and practice breathing.

Now, clasp your hands together behind your buttocks, keeping the elbows slightly bent. Lift the armpits and shoulders up from the front of the chest while squeezing the shoulder blades in toward each other. Inhale as you gently lift the arms away from the buttocks; now exhale and release a bit. Repeat this sequence 5 times.

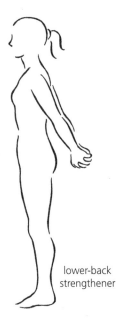

lower-back strengthener

Return to mountain pose and just notice any sensations within the body. Be with yourself. Notice your thoughts, and relax your mind as you prepare for the next posture.

Half Moon

Stand with your feet parallel and hip-width apart. Take a moment to spread your toes and connect your soles with the ground. Press both feet into the ground and lift your knees, feeling your thigh muscles hugging your femurs and connecting to your pelvic muscles. Allow a gentle squeeze, tucking your tailbone in toward your pelvis. Extend your arms out and up overhead as you slowly inhale, interlocking your fingers with your index fingers pointing toward the sky in a steeple-like position. Breathe gently in and out.

On the next inhalation, press your right foot downward as you press your right hip out to

half moon

the side. Extend your interlocked hands toward the left, breathing into the stretch gently. Breathe. Bring your awareness to your inner hip and chest, bringing them forward gently, right shoulder pressing back, as if you are leaning between two panes of glass. Bring your attention to your right side and yield into the stretch. Inhale. As you exhale, release the posture by pressing down into your left sole and return to center.

Next, press into the sole of your left foot, out through your left hip, and up through your arms and hands to the opposite side, reaching to the sky, your head tucked evenly between your arms. Keeping your legs energized, feel that place of stretching and relaxing at the same time. To release, inhale pressing your right leg and sole down into the earth. Come back to center.

As you do this pose, imagine the image of a half moon and its quiet calming beauty on a dark clear night. Feel the effects of the moon and its power on the tide of the ocean.

Triangle Pose

In this pose as in all others, honor the limits of your body. Stand in mountain pose and step your feet 3 to 3½ feet apart. If this feels too challenging, bring your feet closer together. Begin getting centered in this position with your hands on your hips, feet pointing straight ahead.

Breathe, pressing your feet into the ground. In your mind's eye imagine a triangle representing mind, body, and

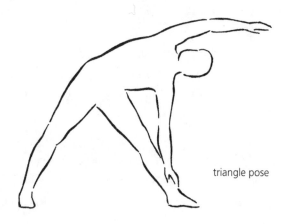

triangle pose

spirit. Be aware of your center of gravity, balancing your weight evenly on each foot, hips facing straight ahead. Relax your pelvis in the center of your hips. As you move into the triangle, keep in mind that you are moving from your center, from the inside out. Breathe from your center, without pushing, and let the breath lead you. Turn your right foot out to your right 90 degrees, and turn your left foot in at a 45-degree angle. Make sure the heel of your right foot is in line with your left instep. Continue to keep your hips facing straight ahead.

Now, as you slowly inhale, lift your arms out to your sides and stretch into your fingertips. Feel your center as you press both feet down, lift your knees, and gaze at the fingers on your right hand. Now begin to reach out through your right fingers as though you want to touch the wall in front of you. As you reach, extend your torso and lower your right hand down onto your right leg; turn your head and gaze at your upper arm.

Bring your hand to whatever place on your leg is comfortable, making sure that there is a straight line of energy from the fingertips of one hand to the fingertips of the other. Engage the breath, allowing your left shoulder to come into alignment with your body, and now focus on bringing the left hip back to center. Invite the breath into your triangle. Let your mind relax into the breath, and focus on balance of mind, body, and spirit. Welcome all that you are in this moment.

To come out of the triangle, reach up through your left hand and arm, inhale, and return to center. Step your feet together, breathe and prepare for the opposite side.

As you enter into triangle pose on your left side, be sure your body is aligned as it was for the triangle pose on the right side, only your left foot will point out 90 degrees and your right foot will point in 45 degrees. Take your time without pressure. Review the sequence of the triangle and give the left side an equal amount of time and energy.

Side-Facing Warrior Pose

Stand in the mountain pose. Focus on the breath. Be aware of supporting your internal organs with the breath. As you inhale, step your legs about three feet apart with your hips facing straight ahead, and exhale. Take a moment to feel your foundation, with your weight evenly distributed, and focus on your breath. Begin to turn your right foot out 90 degrees, and turn your left foot in 45 degrees. Stretch your

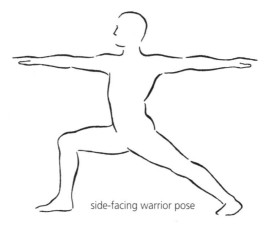

side-facing warrior pose

arms out to your sides at shoulder height. Feel your energy emanating from your abdomen just below your navel down through your legs and feet, and feel grounded. Expand your chest, keeping your torso centered above your pelvis. Make room for your internal organs.

Slowly inhale, and as you exhale bend your right knee so that it is directly over your ankle, forming a right angle. Now continue to breathe down into your abdomen and feel your strength as a warrior. Gaze out over your right hand. Feel your limbs supporting and making room for your internal organs as you breathe slowly. Feel yourself relaxed and, at the same time, expanding, creating space in your joints. Remain in this posture and breathe.

Now straighten your right knee, and return your right foot back so that it is parallel with your left foot. Inhale as you bring your arms to your hips; rest for a moment and breathe normally. Now, repeat the same sequence on the left side.

Slowly lower your body until you are lying down on your abdomen. Be aware of each movement of your body as you come to this position. Take a moment and relax, feeling your body on the ground. Feel the earth supporting your weight, and let go into the breath.

Mind and body are inseparably one.

— Deepak Chopra

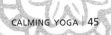

Floor Stretches

Boat Pose

Lying on your abdomen, place either your chin or your forehead on the ground, arms extended forward in front of you, palms facing each other. If you find this too challenging, you may keep your arms down by your sides.

Begin to invite your breath in to your abdomen as you press your pubic bone into the earth. Hold for the count of 5. Release the breath slowly and feel your body relaxing. Feel your connection to the earth. Repeat 2 more times. Be aware of a gradual tightening of your buttock muscles as you press your pubic bone down into the floor.

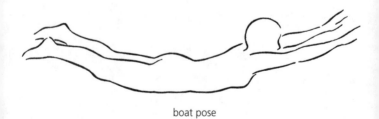

boat pose

On the next inhalation, press your pubic bone down and lift your hands and legs. Extend your arms forward and up, as though you were reaching out to the sky; extend your legs back and up, reaching out through your toes. Keep your head between your arms (unless they are at your sides). Your body will be curved like a boat. Now, breathe evenly and smoothly while holding the posture. When you are ready, inhale, and as you exhale release slowly and gracefully out of the pose.

Breathe, relax your body into the earth, and let go. Feel the wonderful benefits of this pose, such as strengthening your dorsal muscles, legs, and arms; massaging your abdominal organs; and creating space. Feel your strength from the inside out.

Child Pose

As a counter-stretch to the boat pose, move from lying on your abdomen up to a seated position with knees bent, your buttocks resting on your heels. If this is too challenging, place a folded blanket between your heels and your upper thighs. Make it as thick as feels satisfying. This position should not be painful, just a delightful stretch. If you have a knee injury, proceed with caution.

Inhale slowly, and press down into your sitting bones and extend up through the crown of your head. As you exhale,

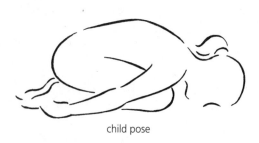

child pose

lift and extend your torso forward across your upper thighs to a resting position with your forehead on the ground. Again, if this posture feels uncomfortable and you feel too much pressure in your head, place a firm pillow or blanket to support your head. Breathe evenly and smoothly, consciously relaxing the muscles in your lower back. Let go and enjoy the child pose. You may want to sway gently from side to side. If you are flexible enough in your arms, bring your hands to rest on your lower spine and feel the support as you rock from side to side. Breathe and let go; enjoy. Come home to yourself.

This pose tranquilizes the whole body while providing a counter-stretch for backward bends, such as the boat pose. It soothes and massages the abdominal organs while increasing flexibility in hips and legs.

Cobra Pose

Return to a belly-down position with your forehead on the ground. Place your palms beneath your shoulders with your elbows close to your body. While keeping your head and hands grounded, inhale, press your pubic bone into the ground, and feel a gradual tightening in your buttock muscles. Hold, exhale, and release.

Next, inhale, press your pubic bone into the ground, and begin to extend your chin, pressing up through the crown of your head. Now, gradually press your palms into the floor and draw your chest forward and up. Relax your shoulders and roll your shoulder blades in toward each other. Listen to your body and concentrate on the breath, slowly inhaling and exhaling. The focus is on lifting and extending the spine while opening the chest.

Press into your palms and feel your strength in your arms. Keep your elbows close to your body. Open and expand your chest. Avoid hyperextending your back body. Let the breath open your heart and lungs. Again, pay attention to your limits, and when you feel that you are ready, inhale, exhale, and gradually release. Return to lying flat, and rest. Slowly come into to the child pose.

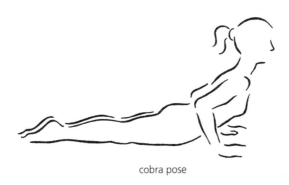

cobra pose

Sphinx Pose

The sphinx pose may be used as an alternate to the cobra pose, or you may enjoy it in addition to the cobra pose.

Lying on your belly, lift your chest and place your elbows just below your shoulders with your forearms parallel to each other and extended forward along the floor. Keep the palms and fingers spread flat on the ground.

Begin pressing your pubic bone into the ground as you activate your inner spine. Invite your breath into your abdomen. Keep your shoulders relaxed, pressing your

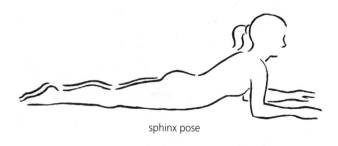

sphinx pose

elbows into the ground. Imagine that you are drawing your upper arms and elbows toward the body. Close your eyes and feel this delightful stretch. Allow the chest to open as you breathe down into the abdomen. Extend back through your toes. Breathe 4 or 5 times while in the sphinx pose.

Release and gently roll over to your back for the next set of delicious stretches.

Leg Stretches

Lie on your back, legs extended, arms down by your sides. Be aware of your alignment. If your neck is hyperextended, you might want to put a folded towel under your head. Feel the support of the ground beneath you. As you lie against the ground, feel the alignment of the mountain pose. Be aware of your energy as you inhale, and as you exhale, let go into the earth.

Bringing your attention to your right leg, bend your knee and wrap your arms around your shin or your upper thigh (under your knee) and interlock your fingers.

Inhale as you bring your thigh closer to your chest. Hold. Exhale. Release. Repeat, coordinating the breath with your movements.

Straighten your leg so that it is perpendicular to the ceiling, and press your heel toward the sky. Place your hands as far up your leg as is comfortable while you rest relaxed on the floor. If your back is strained, bend your left knee with the sole of your left foot flat on the floor.

As you inhale, draw your right leg in toward your chest. Hold for 5 counts. Exhale. Release. Repeat 5 times. End by

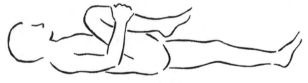

leg stretches

drawing your knee once again into your chest and lifting your head toward your knee. If you want a greater stretch, straighten your left leg along the floor. Always coordinate the breath with the movements. Repeat this sequence with your left leg.

Knee-Down Twist

Lying on your back with both legs extended on the floor, bend your left leg and place the sole of your left foot on your right knee. Roll the left knee toward the right. You can use your right hand on the left knee to bring the knee down toward the floor as far as feels comfortable. Listen once again to your body and honor its limits.

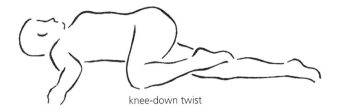

knee-down twist

Extend your left arm straight out from the body, shoulder on the floor. Turn your head to the left and gaze at your left hand.

Breathe into the stretch, and let the breath open your holding. Imagine a gentle hand touching your lumbar spine, and release without pressuring yourself to do more. If you feel pain, you've gone too far; back up and breathe into any sensation you might be experiencing. Coordinate the breath with opening. When you feel ready, release the pose, and come back onto your back.

Before repeating the stretch on the other side, bend your knees to your chest, place one hand on each knee, and make circles. Be aware of massaging your sacral area with the movements. Release your sacral muscles into the floor with the movements. This

knees to chest

should feel relaxing. Notice that this movement is also massaging your abdominal organs.

Now do the knee-down twist on the right side. Be aware of your whole body as you move from the knee-down twist into relaxation.

As you finish this yoga practice, listen to what your body needs. Do what your body is calling for. Take a moment and do your own stretching.

Corpse Pose

If you wish, play some soft relaxing music at this time. You may want to cover your body with a blanket or place an eye pillow over your eyes.

* **Lie on your back,** legs out straight, arms down by your sides with palms facing the sky. Feel free to place a cushion or folded blanket under your knees, if it is more comfortable.

* **Cascade your shoulder blades down your back.** Gently, with kindness toward yourself, move your head from side to side, letting go of any held tension in your neck or other parts of your body.

* **Feel your body and its connection to the earth.** Yield to the earth and feel the effects of your day's yoga practice.

* **Bring your awareness to your breath,** and just notice it without changing it. Let go, and release any holding in your body.

* **Imagine that each breath** is like the waves of the ocean as they embrace the shore, moving and letting go as one joins the other. Feel the earth supporting your whole being and all the miraculous parts of who you are.

* **Embrace your dark and light side** at this moment. If any emotions such as sadness, grief, joy, or anger are present, just breathe into their presence.

* **Let any judgments go.** Honor and mother all of who you are and take in a breath of compassion for all your experiences in life.

* **When your mind begins to wander,** gently bring your attention back to your breath. Feel your connection to life emanating within you. Relax and just be.

* **You have nowhere to go,** nothing to do at this moment. Be aware of taking this experience with you in whatever you do throughout the day, and continue to mother yourself. Let the petals of your practice begin to unfold.

*Within you there is a stillness and sanctuary
to which you can retreat at any time
and be yourself.*

—Herman Hesse, *Siddhartha*

Recommended Reading

Hatha Yoga: The Hidden Language by Swami Sivananda Raddha. Timeless Books, 1995.

Kripalu Yoga Posture Sheets. Kripalu Center for Yoga & Health, 1990.

Yoga: Mind, Body and Spirit: A Return to Wholeness by Donna Farhi. Owl Books, 2000.

Yoga for Woman: Complete Mind and Body Fitness by Paddy O'Brien. HarperCollins, 1991.